KETO CHAFFLE RECIPES 2020

100+ Mouth Watering Low Carb Recipes For Beginners. Bonus: Gluten Free Recipes For Athletes + Anti Aging Recipes For Women Over 50 + Ketogenic Diet Cookbook

Serena Green

© Copyright 2019 by **Serena Green**   All rights reserved.

This document is geared towards providing exact and reliable information with regards to the topic and issue covered. The publication is sold with the idea that the publisher is not required to render accounting, officially permitted, or otherwise, qualified services. If advice is necessary, legal or professional, a practiced individual in the profession should be ordered.

From a Declaration of Principles which was accepted and approved equally by a Committee of the American Bar Association and a Committee of Publishers and Associations.

In no way is it legal to reproduce, duplicate, or transmit any part of this document in either electronic means or in printed format. Recording of this publication is strictly prohibited and any storage of this document is not allowed unless with written permission from the publisher. All rights reserved.

The information provided herein is stated to be truthful and consistent, in that any liability, in terms of inattention or otherwise, by any usage or abuse of any policies, processes, or directions contained within is the solitary and utter responsibility of the recipient reader. Under no circumstances will any legal responsibility or blame be held against the publisher for any reparation, damages, or monetary loss due to the information herein, either directly or indirectly.

Respective authors own all copyrights not held by the publisher.

The information herein is offered for informational purposes solely, and is universal as so. The presentation of the information is without contract or any type of guarantee assurance.

The trademarks that are used are without any consent, and the publication of the trademark is without permission or backing by the trademark owner. All trademarks and brands within this book are for clarifying purposes only and are the owned by the owners themselves, not affiliated with this document

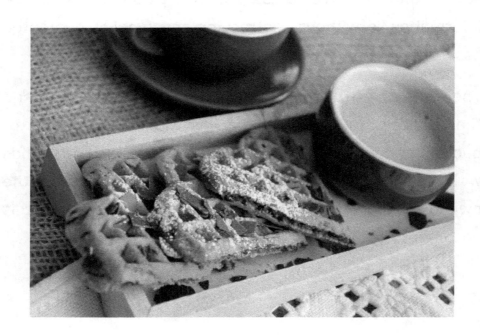

Table of contents

The Meaning Of Chaffle 1

What Is Needed To Prepare A Chaffle 4

How To Prepare A Chaffle 4

The Waffle Tools To Make Easy Keto Chaffles 5

How To Eat Chaffles 6

The Different Type Of Waffle Maker Needed To Make A Chaffle 7

Rules On How To Make The Best Chaffles 8

The Best Keto Chaffle Recipes To Try 13

Keto Chaffle Recipe 13

Rich And Creamy Chaffles Recipe 14

Zucchini Chuffles | Zuffles Recipe 15

Light And Crispy Chaffles Recipe 15

Keto Sausage Ball 16

Fat Head Pizza Crust 17

Chicken Stuffed Avocado 19

Almond Flour Blueberry Pancakes 20

Boston Brown Bread Recipe 21

Keto Cheese Muffins 22

Air Fryer Breaded Chicken Wings 22

One Step Brazilian Pao De Queijo Brazilian Cheese Bread 23

Keto Zucchini Walnut Bread 24

Keto Bread | Nut And Seed Bread 25

One Step Brazilian Pao De Queijo Brazilian Cheese Bread 27

Sweet Cream Truffles 27

Keto Milky Bears| Gummy Bear Recipe 28

Keto Coconut Panna Cotta.. 29

Keto Chocolate Cheesecake Brownies 30

Keto Pie Crust 32

Keto Maple Pecan Blondies...................................... 32

Keto Lasagna 33

Keto Almond Phirni Kheer 34

Tomato Eggplant Soup 34

Hamburger KHEEMA MEATLOAF 35

Weight COOKER LOW CARB WONTONS 36

Keto Chicken Biryani 36

Moment Pot Cauliflower "Macintosh" And Cheese Low Carb 37

Keto Ham And Bean Soup 38

Simple MANGO CARDAMOM PANNACOTTA 39

Smooth SHRIMP SCAMPI 39

Moment POT SPAGHETTI SQUASH 40

Tomato Eggplant Soup 40

Moment POT SAUERKRAUT SOUP RECIPE.................... 41

Chicken And Mushrooms Recipe................................... 42

Keto Shrimp Scampi 42

Essential Indian Curry Recipe | Pressure Cooker Curry Recipe... 43

Chicken Tikka Masala 44

Simple Traditional Keto Chaffle................................... 45

Keto Strawberry Shortcake Chaffle............................ 45

Keto Pumpkin Cheesecake Chaffle............................. 46

Tasty Keto Pizza Chaffle Recipe 46

Pizza Topping 47

Best Oreo Keto Chaffles... 47

Keto Peanut Butter Cup Chaffle 48

Keto Snickerdoodle Chaffle 48

White Bread Keto Chaffle | Wonder Bread Chaffle 50

Best Oreo Keto Chaffles... 50

Keto Chocolate Chip Chaffle Keto Recipe 51

Keto Strawberry Cheesecake Shake 52

Keto Taco Chaffle Recipe (Crispy Taco Shells) 53

Maple Pumpkin Keto Waffle Recipe (Chaffle) 54

Keto Chaffle Breakfast Sandwich 55

Mini Keto Pizza Recipe 55

Sugar-Free Vanilla Buttercream Frosting 56

Keto Blueberry Chaffle 57

Bacon Cheddar Chaffles Recipe 58

Bacon Jalapeno Chaffles Recipe 58

Keto Cauliflower Chaffles Recipe 58

Sandwich Bread Chaffles Recipe 59

Sweet Chaffles Recipes 59

Chocolate Brownie Chaffles 60

Mint Chocolate Broffle (Brownie Waffle) 60

Lemon Pound Cake Chaffles 60

Cream Cheese Carrot Cake Chaffles 61

Cream Cheese Frosting 61

Cinnamon Chaffles 62

Cinnamon Swirl Chaffles 63

Cinnamon Drizzle: 63

Greek Marinated Feta And Olives 64

Air Fryer Peanut Chicken 64

Green Beans With Bacon 65

Keto Buffalo Chicken Casserole.................................. 66

German Red Cabbage.. 66

Maple Pecan Bars With Sea Salt................................. 67

Moment POT VEGETARIAN CHILI 67

Keto Almendrados Cookies | Spanish Almond Keto Cookies
.... 68

Keto Taco 69

Keto Omelet With Goat Cheese And Spinach.............. 69

Chicken And Cheese Quesadilla 70

Gluten Free Sports Nutrition Basics 71

Protein Needs... 71

Carb Requirements 71

Fat Recommendations 72

Gluten Free Recipes For Athletes 73

Almond Blast Protein Shake 73

Chocolate Peanut Butter Protein Balls 74

Tomato Spinach Omelet 75

Quinoa And Asparagus Chicken Salad 76

Turkey Chili 78

Anti-Aging Recipes 80

Edamame With Ground Bonito And Seaweed 80

Korean Pickles.. 81

Pan Fried Food BEEF WITH SPICY HOISIN SAUCE....... 83

Sauteed Kale With Mustard Sauce 85

Sauteed Green Beans With Chilies............................ 87

Shrimp And Celery Salad With Wasabi Mayo.............. 89

Fish Steak With Tomato Relish.................................. 91

Stout Vegetable Soup... 93

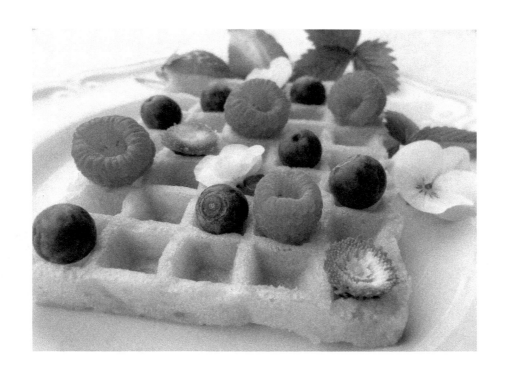

The Meaning Of Chaffle

Chaffles (short for cheddar waffles) are the most recent famous nourishment in the keto world. It's nothing unexpected — the chaffle has a great deal putting it all on the line. This straightforward keto formula is fresh, brilliant dark colored, sans sugar, low-carb, and exceptionally simple to make.

A chaffle, or cheddar waffle, is a keto waffle made with eggs and cheddar. Chaffles are turning into an extremely well known keto/low-carb nibble.

A chaffle is a waffle yet made with a cheddar base. Basically it's obliterated cheddar and an egg mix. Once in for a short time for logically fluffier recipes, it's a cream cheddar base instead of decimated cheddar. It's the a la mode new keto-pleasing bread since it's low in carbs, and it won't spike your insulin levels, causing fat accumulating.

The fundamentals are some combo of egg and cheddar; however, from here, you can riff like wild eyed. You can use an arrangement of cheeses, including cream cheddar, parmesan cheddar, etc. Some incorporate almond flour and flaxseed and getting ready powder, and others don't.

The major recipe for a chaffle contains cheddar, almond flour, and an egg. You consolidate the fixings in an astonish and pour it your waffle maker. Waffle makers are no doubt on the rising right now after this chaffle recipe exploded a couple of days back earlier. I was to some degree suspicious from the beginning intuition there was no possibility this would turn out in the wake of joining everything and pouring the hitter over the waffle. Try to sprinkle the waffle maker really well. The waffle wound up exceptional, and it was firm apparently and fragile in the inside.

You can concoct a chaffle utilizing a waffle iron or smaller than usual waffle producer. The cook time is just a couple of moments, and on the off chance that you cook the chaffle right, you end up with a fresh, gooey, flavorful bread/waffle elective.

Chaffles are turning into somewhat of a furor with supporters of the keto diet. They're less fastidious to make than most keto bread recipes and they're anything but difficult to customize. You can transform the fundamental formula for a chaffle into your own creation, running from flavorful to sweet and anything in the middle. You can likewise change the sort of cheddar you use, delivering significant changes in the flavor and surface of the chaffle. Cheddar and mozzarella cheddar are the two most regular decisions, yet you can likewise include parmesan, cream cheddar, or whatever other cheddar that melts well.

The most fundamental clarification of a Chaffle is that it's an extraordinary bread elective when on the keto diet. It copies the vibe of a waffle however Keto clients have been utilizing Chaffles in a wide range of recipes from sandwiches to sweets. There are a huge amount of Keto Chaffle Recipes out there.

The first chaffle formula starting point is obscure. Be that as it may, what a chaffle is – well, it's Keto enchantment in your mouth. It's a low carb waffle that works AWESOME for filling your requirement for bread. It just takes a couple of fixings, can be made in merely minutes and is made in a waffle creator.

It's made with cheddar, so get it? At the point when you work cheddar and waffle – you get chaffle (and you additionally get enchantment.) Well enough with the back story. Since you realize what this keto nourishment is, how about we make one and let you see with your own eyes how astounding this keto waffle is.

What Is Needed To Prepare A Chaffle

- 1 tremendous egg
- 1/2 c. Cheddar
- 2 tablespoons of almond flour

How To Prepare A Chaffle

There are a few hints, techniques and approaches you'll need to know to make your chaffles particularly fresh.

Most importantly, don't eat your chaffles directly out of the waffle iron. They'll be wet and eggy from the outset, however on the off chance that you let them sit for 3-4 minutes, they'll fresh right up.

Second, for extra fresh chaffles, you can include an additional layer of destroyed cheddar (or another cheddar that gets firm, similar to parmesan) to the two sides of the waffle producer's surface. Set out the destroyed cheddar, pour in the hitter, put more cheddar on top, and afterward cook the chaffle typically. You'll wind up with firm, sautéed bits of cheddar installed in the outside of the chaffle.

Everyone is going looney tunes, asking, "How might I make these?!" This is the game plan The principal recipe on what and how. The fundamental equation consolidates crushed cheddar and an egg; however, there are tremendous measures of add-ins you can use to change the flavor! You will make a direct chaffle hitter and cook it in a waffle maker!

To make a chaffle equation, you will fundamentally join two or three fixings and cook it in a waffle maker to make a perfect work of art everyone will value!

1. Preheat your waffle maker if it requires preheating.
2. Whisk together the egg, cheddar, almond flour, and setting up the soda pop in a bowl until all-around joined.
3. Shower the waffle maker with a cooking sprinkle and pour the chaffle player over the waffle maker. Close and let the waffle for 3 to 4 minutes. My waffle maker has it's own customized clock setting.
4. Remove the waffle from the waffle press and welcome it.

The Waffle Tools To Make Easy Keto Chaffles

A standard waffle creator will deliver a chaffle that appears as though the universally adored round solidified toaster waffles, which is flawless as keto bread for sandwiches, a bun for burgers, or even a shell for tacos. One famous brand is the Dash smaller than expected waffle creator, which is entirely reasonable and makes slender, fresh chaffles.

A Belgian waffle creator makes thicker waffles with profound scores. That is incredible for typical waffle-production, however it isn't perfect for chaffles. They end up less fresh, with a greater amount of an omelet-like consistency. Your most logical option is to get a standard waffle producer.

How To Eat Chaffles

There are a great deal of famous approaches to eat chaffles.

- Plain. Chaffles are incredible all alone as a morning meal nourishment. You can serve them up close by bacon, eggs, avocado, and other standard keto breakfast passage.
- Keto chaffle sandwich. Make two chaffles and use them as bread for your preferred sandwich. Chaffles are extraordinary as the bread for BLTs, turkey clubs, breakfast sandwiches, or some other keto-accommodating sandwich.
- Chaffle dessert. Attempt one of the sweet chaffle varieties recorded underneath and present with keto maple syrup or your most loved keto frozen yogurt.

The Different Type Of Waffle Maker Needed To Make A Chaffle

By far most genuinely like to use a Dash Mini Waffle Maker; however, you can use any waffle maker you have. There is a wide scope of waffle makers. Honestly, you in all likelihood have one in the back of your kitchen organizers that you haven't used in quite a while. Most by far who don't have a waffle maker may even find one at a Goodwill or Salvation Army. There's no absence of these helpful kitchen gadgets in these reused stores.

The Various Types Of Basic Keto Chaffle Recipes

Keto Chaffle Recipes eBook Cookbook for beginners 2020, includes delicious and appealing keto recipes for each flavor palette.

1. Basic Chaffle Recipes
2. Savory Chaffle Recipes
3. Sweet Chaffle Recipes
4. Chaffle Cake Recipes

Various Cheeses

Cheddar, mozzarella, parmesan, cream cheddar, colby jack — any cheddar that melts well will work with a chaffle. Distinctive cheddar produce various flavors and somewhat various surfaces. Attempt a couple and locate your top choice.

Sweet Chaffles

Utilize a nonpartisan cheddar like mozzarella or cream cheddar, at that point include a touch of your most loved keto sugar to the hitter before you cook it. You can likewise chocolate chips or low-sugar fruits like blueberries or strawberries. Top with keto frozen yogurt or keto whipped cream for a delectable chaffle dessert.

Exquisite Chaffles

Include exquisite fixings like herbs and flavors to your chaffle. For a pizza chaffle, include oregano, garlic powder, and diced pepperoni in the hitter, with tomato sauce and additional cheddar on top. Or on the other hand you could utilize cream cheddar and add everything bagel flavoring to the player for an everything bagel chaffle. Present with more cream cheddar on top, tricks, onions, and smoked salmon.

Rules On How To Make The Best Chaffles

1. Tolerance. That is the best tip. They don't take long, yet if you need a new keto waffle, you are just should be to some degree patient and let it take the 5-7 minutes that it takes to new up.

Precisely when you trust it's done? Permit it one greater minute or two. Make an effort not to flood.

2. Layering. In the event that you're making a chaffle with cheddar, the best way to deal with do this is to layer cheddar at the base, pour in a tablespoon or so of egg, and a short time later top with cheddar again. It's the firm cheddar on the base and top that will make them new.

3. Shallow waffles. If you need new waffles, the shallower the waffle iron, the more straightforward/faster it is to new up the chaffle.

4. No over-burdening. Stuffed chaffle makers... well, they flood clearly. Which makes colossal destruction! So when in doubt, under fill rather than pressing. Near 1/4 cup of TOTAL fixings in a steady progression.

5. Crush it. I've thought about others using press bottles so they can get just a little egg into the small scale waffle maker.

6. Simple cleanup. I like to use a wet paper towel when the waffle iron is warm, to make cleanup straightforward. Not hot, however, obviously! Essentially warm.

7. Brush it. I've found toothbrush works outstandingly to clean between the waffle iron

teeth. You can in like manner endeavor this wipe cleaner, which I also use to clean the little region on the edge of my Instant Pot.

8. No looking. I can tell you from LOTS of individual experience, that opening the waffle iron at normal interims "just to check" doesn't hep the chaffle cook any speedier. Your most consistent choice is to not using any and all means open it for 4-5 minutes.

9. No steaming. on the off chance that you're using the Dash small, the little blue light goes out when it's commonly cooked, yet most importantly, the chaffle stops steaming to such a degree. That is a better than average sign that it's done.

10. Get hot. Hold up until the waffle iron is hot before you incorporate fixings, and they're essentially less slanted to adhere and a lot easier to clean up.

11. Tangle it. Alright, so about that flood. I do find that it unfolds more routinely than I may need! One thing that has made cleanup more straightforward for me has been to put a silicone trivet underneath.

12. Cut or shred. I understand most recipes out there suggest demolished cheddar, yet I have better karma with the slimmest cut of cheddar I can buy. I find it crisps essentially speedier.

13. Not really eggy. If you find your chaffles too eggy, use egg white as opposed to the whole egg.
14. Not really gooey. In case you need them to taste less gooey, endeavor mozzarella cheddar.
15. Fresh Cooling. License the chaffles to cool before eating. They get crisper as they cool, so take the necessary steps not to stuff the hot chaffle into your mouth right away.
16. Make parts. Make enough to share, and everyone will require them, whether or not they're keto or not.

Chaffles Nutrition and Carb Count

You'll get two chaffles out of an enormous egg and about a large portion of a cup of cheddar. Contingent upon the cheddar you use, your calories and net carb check will change a tad. Yet, as a rule, expecting you utilize genuine, entire milk cheddar like cheddar or mozzarella (rather than cream cheddar or American cheddar), chaffles are totally sans carb. A normal serving size of two chaffles contains generally:

- 300 calories
- 0g all out carbs
- 0g net carbs
- 20g protein

- 23g fat

As should be obvious, chaffles are about as keto as a formula can be: high-fat, high-protein, and zero-carb. They even work on the flesh eater diet, if you eat cheddar.

The Best Keto Chaffle Recipes To Try

Including recipes for some work of art, high-carb top picks that have been adjusted to be "fat bombs," which help keep your macros in balance, just as keep you from desiring every one of the things you, for the most part, can't eat when you're attempting to get more fit.

A considerable amount of the in excess of 200 recipes require close to 10 to 15 minutes of planning time, and they taste as scrumptious and liberal as they sound—what about Chocolate Peanut Butter Pops, Mocha Cheesecake, or Almond Butter Bombs?

Keto Chaffle Recipe

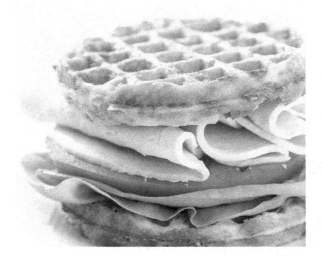

Keto chaffles are the most recent new rage! The entire formula is just 3 net carbs all out.

INGREDIENTS

- 1 huge egg
- 1/2 c. Cheddar
- 2 tablespoons of almond flour

Rich And Creamy Chaffles Recipe

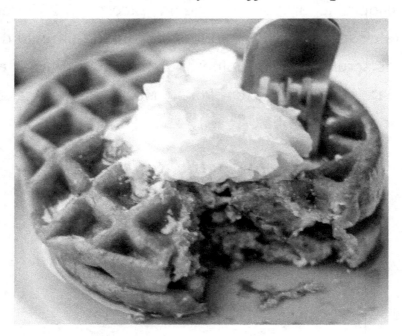

- 2 eggs
- 1 cup destroyed mozzarella
- 2 tablespoons almond flour
- 2 tablespoons cream cheddar
- 3/4 Tbsp. preparing power

- 3 tablespoons water (discretionary)
- Makes 6 waffles.

Zucchini Chuffles | Zuffles Recipe

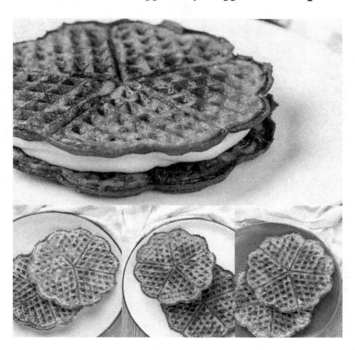

- 1 little zucchini, ground
- 1 egg
- 1 tablespoon parmesan
- Small bunch of destroyed mozzarella
- Basil and pepper to taste
- Mix all together and cook in a full-size waffle producer.
- Makes 2 full-size waffles and a meager zaffle.

Light And Crispy Chaffles Recipe

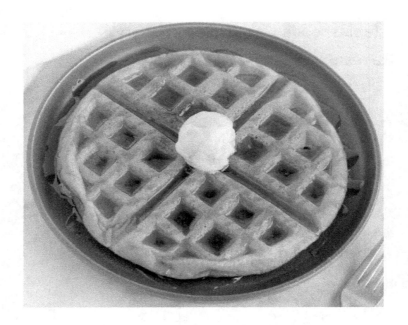

- 1 egg
- 1/3 cup cheddar
- 1/4 Tbsp. heating powder
- 1/2 Tbsp. ground flaxseed
- Shredded parmesan cheddar on top and base.
- Stir and cook in a mini waffle iron until fresh.

Keto Sausage Ball

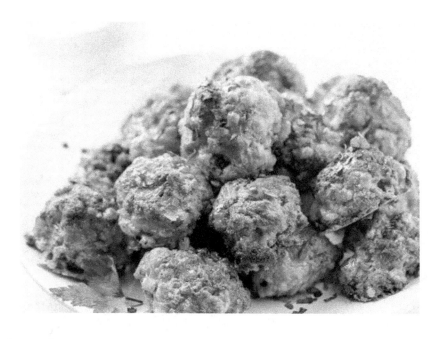

Portrayal

Keto Sausage Balls just contain four straightforward ingredients and make an extraordinary canapé or bite. They just contain 1 net carb and can without much of a stretch fit into your low carb or keto way of life.

INGREDIENTS

- 2 cups of almond flour
- 2 cups of cheddar
- 1 pound of pork wiener
- 8 oz of cream cheddar

Fat Head Pizza Crust

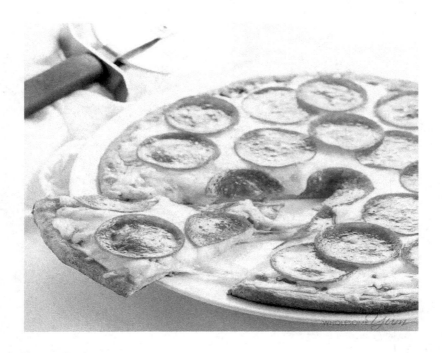

INGREDIENTS

- 1 1/2 cups destroyed mozzarella
- 3/4 cup almond flour
- 2 tablespoons of cream cheddar, cubed
- 1 egg
- garlic powder, onion powder, and blended herbs for flavoring *see notes

Chicken Stuffed Avocado

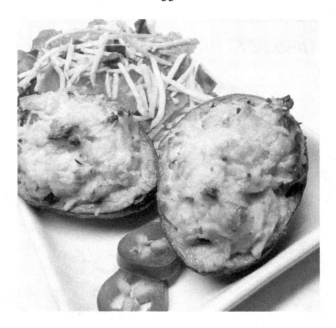

Portrayal

Wild ox Chicken Stuffed Avocado is a brisk formula utilizing stovetop bison chicken plunge and avocados. Making wild ox chicken plunge is extremely simple utilizing a stovetop too.

INGREDIENTS

- 2 5 oz jars of chicken, depleted
- 2 tablespoons of whipped cream cheddar
- 2 tsp of dry Ranch flavoring blend
- ¼ cup of sans fat cheddar (utilize full fat with keto or low carb)

- 2 tablespoons of Frank's Buffalo Wing Sauce
- 1 medium avocado

Almond Flour Blueberry Pancakes

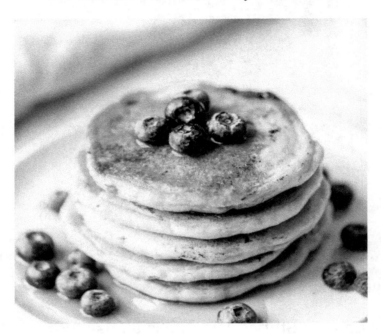

Depiction

Basic almond flour flapjacks made with just 6 ingredients. 2 net carbs per hotcake!

INGREDIENTS

- 2 huge eggs
- ⅓ cup unsweetened almond milk
- 1 Tbsp. vanilla concentrate
- 1 ¼ cup fine almond flour (utilized Bob's, Red Mill)
- ¼ Tbsp. preparing pop

- Touch of salt
- Spread for lubing the skillet

Boston Brown Bread Recipe

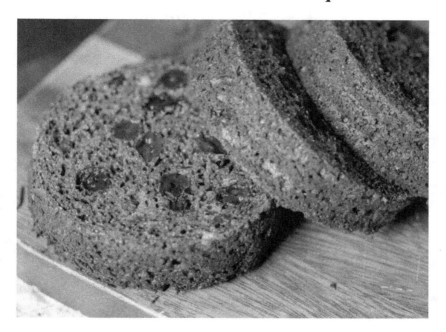

Ingredients

- 1 Egg
- 1 cup buttermilk, or 1 cup milk with 1 tablespoon vinegar blended in
- 1/4 cup Molasses
- 1/4 cup Sugar
- 1 tablespoon Oil
- 1.5 cups Whole Wheat Flour
- 1/2 cup Cornmeal
- 2 Tbsp.s Baking Powder

- 1 Tbsp. Ground Allspice
- 1/2 cup slashed pecans
- 1/4 cup Raisins

Keto Cheese Muffins

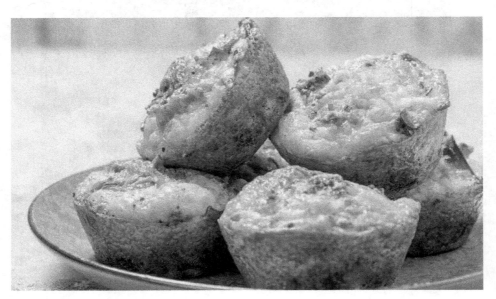

Ingredients

- Vegetable oil for lubing the skillet
- 1 cup (112 g) Superfine Almond Flour
- 1/2 cup (85 g) Black Chia Seeds
- 2 Tbsp.s (2 Tbsp.s) Baking Powder
- 1/2 Tbsp. (118.29 g) granulated garlic
- 4 enormous (4 huge) Eggs
- 1/4 cup (56.75 g) softened margarine
- 1/2 cup (56.5 g) ground cheddar

Air Fryer Breaded Chicken Wings

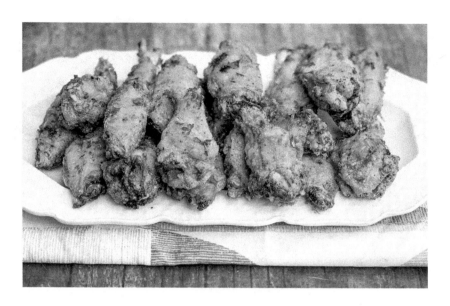

Ingredients

- 1 pound (453.59 g) chicken wings
- 3 tablespoons (3 tablespoons) Vegetable Oil
- 1/2 cup (62.5 g) All-Purpose Flour
- 1/2 Tbsp. (0.5 Tbsp.) Smoked Paprika
- 1/2 Tbsp. (0.5 Tbsp.s) Garlic Powder
- 1/2 Tbsp. (0.5 Tbsp.) Salt
- 1/2 Tbsp. (0.5 Tbsp.s) naturally squashed peppercorn

One Step Brazilian Pao De Queijo Brazilian Cheese Bread

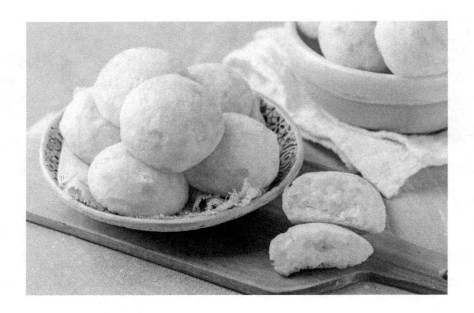

Ingredients

- 1 cup (244 g) Whole Milk
- 1/2 cup (112 g) Oil
- 1 Tbsp. (1 Tbsp.) Salt
- 2 cups (240 g) Tapioca Flour
- 2 (2) Eggs
- 1.5 cups (150 g) destroyed parmesan cheddar

Keto Zucchini Walnut Bread

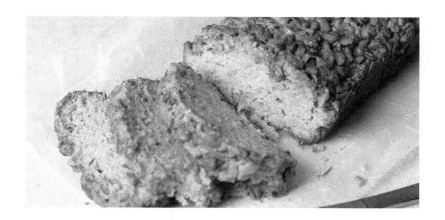

Need to make a Keto Zucchini Bread, you'll be super eager to eat and serve to other people? This formula with pecans is great!

Ingredients

- 1/2 cup (0.5 g) Truvia
- 3 (3) Eggs
- 1/2 cup (109 g) Ghee or Oil
- 1.5 cups (168 g) Superfine Almond Flour
- 1/2 cups (60 g) coconut flour
- 1 Tbsp. (1 Tbsp.) Baking Powder
- 1 Tbsp. (1 Tbsp.) Baking Soda
- 1/2 Tbsp. (0.5 Tbsp.s) Ground Cinnamon
- 1/4 Tbsp. Ground Nutmeg
- 1/2 cup (250 g) Unsweetened Almond Milk
- 2 cups (248 g) destroyed zucchini
- 1 cup (117 g) cleaved pecans

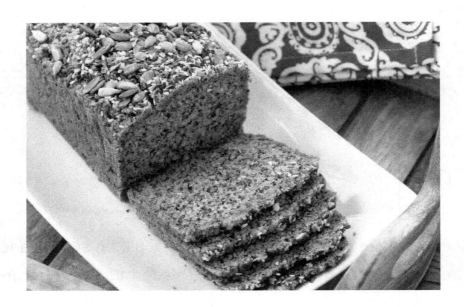

Ingredients

3 cups blended nuts and seeds left entire for instance

- 1/2 cup (61.5 g) pistachios
- 1/2 cup (71.5 g) almonds
- 1/2 cup (84 g) flaxseed
- 1/2 cup (58.5 g) pecans
- 1/2 cup (75 g) Sesame Seeds
- 1/2 cup (64.5 g) cashews

Different ingredients

- 3 (3) Eggs
- 1/4 cup (56 ml) Oil
- 1/3 tsp (0.33 tsp) Salt

One Step Brazilian Pao De Queijo Brazilian Cheese Bread

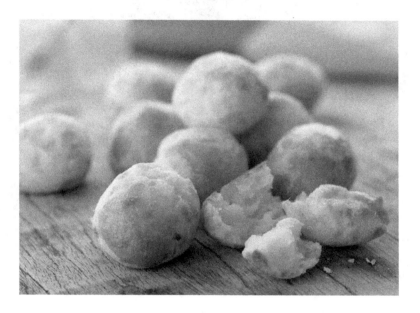

Ingredients

- 1 cup (244 g) Whole Milk
- 1/2 cup (112 g) Oil
- 1 Tbsp. (1 Tbsp.) Salt
- 2 cups (240 g) Tapioca Flour
- 2 (2) Eggs
- 1.5 cups (150 g) destroyed parmesan cheddar

Sweet Cream Truffles

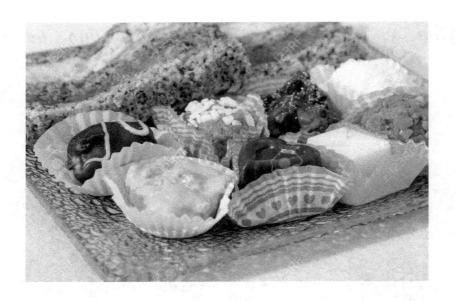

Ingredients

For the Truffle Center

- 2 cups (476 g) Heavy Whipping Cream
- 1/2 cup (91 g) powdered Swerve
- For the Chocolate Coating
- 2 ounces (56.7 g) Sugar-Free Chocolate Chips
- 1 tablespoon (1 tablespoon) Butter

Keto Milky Bears| Gummy Bear Recipe

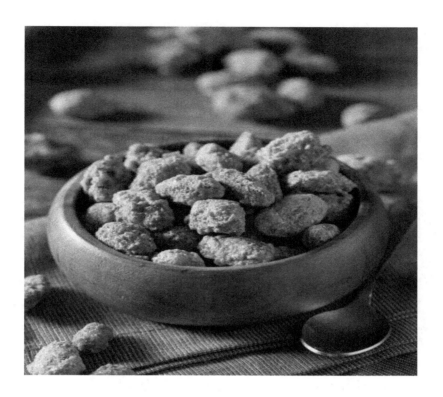

These Keto Milky Bears are a fabulous sweet treat that won't take you out of ketosis. They're low carb, without gluten thus great you can't simply eat one! Obviously superior to normal keto sticky bears.

Ingredients

- 1 13.5 ounces (1) Full-Fat Coconut Milk
- 2 bundles (2) unflavored gelatin, (3 tablespoons)
- 1/4 cup (62.5 g) Water
- 3 tablespoons (3 tablespoons) Truvia
- 2-3 drops (2) Pandan Extract

Keto Coconut Panna Cotta

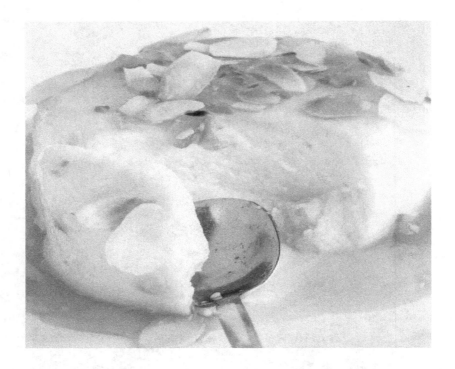

This straightforward Coconut Panna Cotta formula so sweet, smooth, and yummy that it will get one of your go-to pastries! Also, it's low carb and dairy-free!

Ingredients

- 1/2 cup cold water
- 1 bundle unflavored gelatin, 1/4 oz or 2.5 Tbsp.s
- 13.5 ounces Full-Fat Coconut Milk
- 1/8 cup Truvia
- 1 Tbsp. unadulterated vanilla concentrate or coconut extricate

Keto Chocolate Cheesecake Brownies

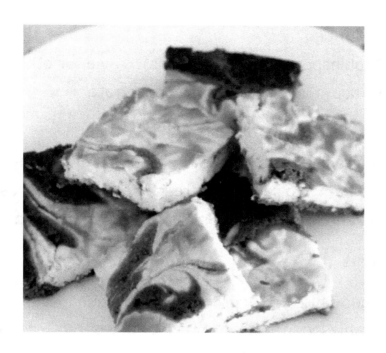

These Keto Chocolate Cheesecake Brownies are a chocolate cheesecake darlings dream! They're so acceptable you won't have the option to tell their low carb!

Ingredients

For the Brownie Batter

- 1/2 cup (90 g) Sugar-Free Chocolate Chips
- 1/2 cup (113.5 g) Butter
- 3 (3) Eggs
- 1/4 cup (0.25 g) Truvia, or other sugar
- 1 Tbsp. (1 Tbsp.) vanilla concentrate
- For the Cheesecake Batter
- 8 ounces (226.8 g) Cream Cheese, cubed and relaxed

- 1 (1) Egg
- 3 tablespoons (3 tablespoons) Truvia, or other sugar
- 1 Tbsp. (1 Tbsp.) vanilla concentrate

Keto Pie Crust

This 3-ingredient pat out Keto Pie Crust formula is a keto dieter's dream! No compelling reason to make crustless pies so as to keep it low carb. It's totally keto and vegan.

Ingredients

- 1 cup (112 g) Superfine Almond Flour
- 2 tablespoons (2 tablespoons) powdered Swerve
- 1/4 cup (54.5 g) Melted Coconut Oil

Keto Maple Pecan Blondies

These Keto Maple Pecan Blondies are the ideal sweet treat to fulfill your sweet tooth. They're wonderfully rich and shockingly low carb!

Ingredients

- 1 cup (112 g) Superfine Almond Flour
- 1/4 cup (30 g) coconut flour
- 2 Tbsp.s (2 Tbsp.s) Baking Powder
- 1/2 cup (91 g) Swerve
- 1/2 cup (113.5 g) Butter, softened
- 3 (3) Eggs
- 1 Tbsp. (1 Tbsp.) maple separate

- 3/4 cup (87.75 g) slashed pecans

Keto Lasagna

Make this simple Keto Lasagna formula in your air fryer utilizing zucchini rather than conventional pasta noodles. It's so acceptable you won't miss the pasta!

Ingredients

- 1 cup marinara sauce
- 1 zucchini, cut into long, flimsy cuts
- For Meat Layer
- 1 cup finely slashed yellow onion
- 1 Tbsp. Minced Garlic
- 1/2 pound-mass hot or mellow Italian frankfurter
- 1/2 cup ricotta cheddar
- 1/2 cup destroyed mozzarella cheddar
- 1/2 cup destroyed parmesan,, isolated
- 1 Egg
- 1/2 Tbsp. Garlic, minced
- 1/2 Tbsp. Italian Seasoning
- 1/2 Tbsp. Ground Black Pepper

Keto Almond Phirni Kheer

This Keto Almond Phirni Kheer is a heavenly Indian pastry formula that you're going to experience passionate feelings for! In addition, it is tasty, it's low carb as well!

Ingredients
- 3/4 cup (178.5 g) Heavy Whipping Cream
- 1 cup (250 g) Unsweetened Almond Milk
- 1/2 cup (56 g) Superfine Almond Flour
- 2 tablespoons (2 tablespoons) Truvia
- 1/2-1 Tbsp. (0.5 Tbsp.s) Ground Cardamom
- 2-3 (2) Saffron Strands, squashed

Tomato Eggplant Soup

This is such an incredible vegan Tomato Eggplant Soup formula! Empty everything into your Instant Pot, and you'll have a bowl of great Mediterranean soup for supper in less than 30 minutes.

Ingredients
- 3 tablespoons Oil
- 2 tablespoons Minced Garlic
- 4 cups Eggplant, hacked
- 2 cups Tomatoes, hacked, or 1 14.5 ounce canned tomatoes, depleted
- 1 cup Onion, hacked

- 1 cup chime pepper, cleaved
- 1/2 cup Water
- 1 Tbsp. salt
- 1 Tbsp. Ground Black Pepper
- For Finishing
- 1/4 cup Basil, hacked

Hamburger KHEEMA MEATLOAF

Tired of normal meatloaf? Can't manage one more night of tacos to go through that ground hamburger? Make proper acquaintance with air fryer keto Indian Kheema meatloaf! Appreciate Indian food in a manner you may be comfortable with by making this Beef Kheema Meatloaf in your Air Fryer.

Ingredients

- 1 lb Lean Ground Beef
- 2 Eggs
- 1 cup Onion, diced
- 1/4 cup Cilantro, hacked
- 1 tbsp minced ginger
- 1 tbsp Minced Garlic
- 2 tsp Garam Masala
- 1 tsp Salt
- 1 tsp Turmeric
- 1 tsp cayenne
- 1/2 tsp Ground Cinnamon

- 1/8 tsp Ground Cardamom

Weight COOKER LOW CARB WONTONS

Make these low carb wontons in your Instant pot, for the most delicate and succulent low carb wontons you've at any point had. Make these wontons without any wrappers, yet the entirety of the flavor of customary wontons.

Ingredients

- 1 pound (453.59 g) ground pork
- 1/4 cup (25 g) Green Onions, green and white parts blended
- 1/4 cup (4 g) Chopped Cilantro or Parsley
- 2 Tbsp.s (2 Tbsp.s) Soy Sauce
- 1 Tbsp. (1 Tbsp.) Oyster sauce
- 1 Tbsp. (1 Tbsp.) Ground Black Pepper
- ½ Tbsp. (0.5 Tbsp.) Salt
- 1 tablespoon (1 tablespoon) minced ginger
- 1 tablespoon (1 tablespoon) Minced Garlic
- 2 (2) Eggs

Keto Chicken Biryani

This Low Carb Chicken Biryani formula is Low-Carb Indian Food at it's ideal. Cauliflower and ground chicken make up this fiery, heavenly low carb formula.

Ingredients

For Chicken

- 1 Tbsp. Ghee
- 1 pound Ground Chicken
- 1 Tbsp. salt
- 1/2 Tbsp. Turmeric
- 1 Tbsp. Garam Masala
- 1/2 Tbsp. Ground Coriander
- 1/4 Tbsp. Ground Cumin

Vegetables

- 1 Tbsp. Ghee
- 1 Red Onion, cut meager
- 1 Jalapeño pepper, diced
- 1 Tbsp. ginger-garlic glue, (or 1/2 Tbsp.s minced garlic, 1/2 Tbsp.s minced ginger)
- 1/2 cup Water
- 1/2 cup Cilantro, slashed
- 1/4 cup mint leaves, slashed
- 2 cups cauliflower, riced

Moment Pot Cauliflower "Macintosh" And Cheese Low Carb

Moment Pot Low Carb Keto Cauliflower and Cheese is a velvety, delightful side dish that you can make in your weight cooker for a definitive low carb comfort food!

Ingredients

- 2 cups (214 g) cauliflower, riced
- 2 tablespoon (2 tablespoons) Cream Cheese
- 1/2 cup (56.5 g) destroyed sharp cheddar
- 1/2 Tbsp. (0.5 Tbsp.) Salt
- 1/2 Tbsp. (0.5 Tbsp.s) Ground Black Pepper

Keto Ham And Bean Soup

No compelling reason to miss beans on a low carb diet. This Keto Ham and Bean Soup formula utilize a mystery, keto bean substitute that preferences simply like the genuine article.

Ingredients

- 1 cup (186 g) dried dark soybeans, doused to yield 2 cups beans
- 1 cup (160 g) onions, slashed
- 1 cup (101 g) slashed celery
- 4 cloves (4 cloves) Minced Garlic
- 1 Tbsp. (1 Tbsp.) Dried Oregano
- .5 to 1 Tbsp. salt
- 1 Tbsp. (1 Tbsp.) Cajun Seasoning
- 1 Tbsp. (1 Tbsp.) Liquid Smoke
- 2 Tbsp.s (2 Tbsp.s) Tony Chachere's universally handy flavoring

- 1 Tbsp. (1 Tbsp.) Louisiana Hot sauce
- 1 (1) substantial ham bone or 2 smoked ham sells
- 2 cups (280 g) slashed ham
- 2 cups (16.91 floz) Water

Simple Mango Cardamom Pannacotta

Low Carb Panna Cotta sets up rapidly and is a reviving summer dessert. Delicious, rich panna cotta joined with sweet mango.

Ingredients

- 1 tablespoon (1 tablespoon) unflavored gelatin
- 2 cups (488 g) Fairlife entire milk, (separated)
- 1 cup (165 g) mango
- 1 cup (238 g) Heavy Whipping Cream
- 1/2 cup (91 g) Swerve, or other sugar
- 1 Tbsp. (1 Tbsp.) Ground Cardamom

Smooth SHRIMP SCAMPI

Simple Low Carb Keto Creamy Shrimp Scampi from your moment pot or weight cooker, this one cooks quick! Put it over some low carb noodles for a snappy supper.

Ingredients

- 2 tablespoons Butter
- 1 pound Shrimp, solidified
- 4 cloves Garlic, minced

- 1/4-1/2 Tbsp.s Red Pepper Flakes
- 1/2 Tbsp.s Smoked Paprika
- 2 cups Carbanada low carb pasta, (uncooked)
- 1 cup Chicken Broth
- 1/2 cup Half and Half
- 1/2 cup Parmesan Cheese
- Salt, to taste
- Ground Black Pepper, to taste

Moment POT SPAGHETTI SQUASH

When you make Spaghetti squash in the Instant pot, you will never make it another way. Eight minutes under tension, without cutting the squash, and you have the ideal low carb or veggie lover side dish.

Ingredients

- 1 Large Spaghetti Squash
- 1.5 cups Water, for the Instant Pot

Tomato Eggplant Soup

This is such an extraordinary vegan Tomato Eggplant Soup formula! Empty everything into your Instant Pot, and you'll have a magnificent Mediterranean soup for supper in less than 30 minutes.

Ingredients

- 3 tablespoons Oil

- 2 tablespoons Minced Garlic
- 4 cups Eggplant, slashed
- 2 cups Tomatoes, slashed, or 1 14.5 ounce canned tomatoes, depleted
- 1 cup Onion, slashed
- 1 cup ringer pepper, cleaved
- 1/2 cup Water
- 1 Tbsp. salt
- 1 Tbsp. Ground Black Pepper

Moment Pot Sauerkraut Soup Recipe

Utilize your Instant Pot to make this flavorful, low-carb Sauerkraut Soup formula! It's a simple dump and cooks formula that cooks in a short time.

Ingredients

- 1 cup dried cannellini beans, drenched medium-term and depleted
- 14 oz smoked frankfurters, cut down the middle longwise, and afterward cut into 1-inch pieces
- 1 cup sauerkraut with brackish water
- 3 Bay Leaves
- 1 cup onions, slashed
- 1 tablespoon Minced Garlic
- 1 Tbsp. Salt
- 1 Tbsp. Ground Black Pepper

- 4 cups Water

Chicken And Mushrooms Recipe

If you need to make a Chicken and Mushrooms Recipe, however, would prefer not to utilize canned soup, have I got only the thing for you! It's Keto and Instant Pot also!

Ingredients

- 2 tablespoons (2 tablespoons) Butter
- 1 cup (160 g) Sliced Onions
- 6 (6) Garlic Cloves, cut slender
- 1 cup (186 g) Mushrooms, cut into quarters
- 1 lb (453.59 g) Boneless Skinless Chicken Thighs
- 4 cups (120 g) infant spinach
- 2 tablespoons (2 tablespoons) Water
- 1 Tbsp.ful of Dried Thyme, or 3-4 sprigs crisp thyme
- 1 Tbsp. (1 Tbsp.) Salt
- 1 Tbsp.ful of Ground Black Pepper
- For Finishing
- 1/2 cup (119 g) Heavy Whipping Cream
- 1 tablespoon (1 tablespoon) lemon juice

Keto Shrimp Scampi

8 minutes from beginning to end to make this air fryer keto low carb shrimp scampi. So easy to make, so heavenly, you will have a hard time believing it.

Ingredients

- 4 tablespoons (4 tablespoons) Butter
- 1 tablespoon (1 tablespoon) lemon juice
- 1 tablespoon (1 tablespoon) Minced Garlic
- 2 Tbsp.s (2 Tbsp.s) Red Pepper Flakes
- 1 tablespoon (1 tablespoon) hacked chives, or 1 Tbsp. dried chives
- 1 tablespoon (1 tablespoon) hacked crisp basil, or 1 Tbsp. dried basil
- 2 tablespoons of Chicken Stock, (or white wine)
- 1 lb (453.59 g) defrosted shrimp, (21-25 check)

Essential Indian Curry Recipe | Pressure Cooker Curry Recipe

This Basic Indian Curry is a tasty customary Indian curry formula made in the Instant Pot! This curry formula is low-carb and stuffed with Indian flavor.

Ingredients

- 1 pound (453.59 g) Boneless Pork Shoulder, diced into 2 inch 3D squares
- 1.5 cups (240 g) onions, hacked
- 1 cup (242 g) Canned Tomatoes, undrained
- 1 tablespoon (1 tablespoon) Minced Garlic
- 1 tablespoon minced ginger

- 2 Tbsp.s (2 Tbsp.s) Garam Masala, separated
- 1 Tbsp. (1 Tbsp.) Salt
- 1 Tbsp. (1 Tbsp.) Turmeric
- 1/4-1 Tbsp. (0.25 Tbsp.) Cayenne
- 2 tablespoons (2 tablespoons) Water

Chicken Tikka Masala

Make simple, real Chicken Tikka Masala comfortable in your Instant Pot or weight cooker! It's by a wide margin the simplest method to make Chicken Tikka Masala.

Ingredients

Marinate the chicken

- 1 ½ pound (680.39 g) Boneless Skinless Chicken Thighs, (bosom or thighs), cut into enormous pieces
- ½ cups (100 g) Greek Yogurt
- 4 cloves (4 cloves) Garlic, minced
- 2 Tbsp.s (2 Tbsp.s) minced ginger, minced
- ½ Tbsp. (0.5 Tbsp.) Turmeric
- ¼ Tbsp. (0.25 Tbsp.) Cayenne
- ½ Tbsp. (0.5 Tbsp.s) Smoked Paprika, for shading and a somewhat smoky taste
- 1 Tbsp. (1 Tbsp.) Salt
- 1 Tbsp. (1 Tbsp.) Garam Masala
- 1/2 Tbsp. (0.5 Tbsp.s) Ground Cumin

- 1 Tbsp. (1 Tbsp.) Liquid Smoke, (overlook if inaccessible)

Simple Traditional Keto Chaffle

INGREDIENTS

- 1 Egg
- 1/2 cup Shredded Cheddar Cheese

Directions

- Preheat mini waffle creator.
- In a cucp, whisk the egg until beaten.
- Add destroyed cheddar and mix to consolidate.
- When the waffle creator is warmed, cautiously pour 1/2 of the hitter in the waffle producer and close the top. Permit to cook for 3-5 minutes.
- Carefully expel from the waffle producer and put in a safe spot for 2-3 minutes to fresh up.
- Repeat guidelines again for the second chaffle.

Keto Strawberry Shortcake Chaffle

INGREDIENTS

- 1 Egg
- 1 tbsp Heavy Whipping Cream
- 1 tsp Coconut Flour
- 2 tbsp Lakanto Golden Sweetener (Use butter together for 20% off)

- 1/2 tsp Cake Batter Extract
- 1/4 tsp Baking powder

Keto Pumpkin Cheesecake Chaffle

INGREDIENTS

PUMPKIN CHAFFLE

- 1 Egg
- 1/2 cup Mozzarella Cheese
- 1 1/2 tbsp Pumpkin Puree (100% pumpkin)
- 1 tbsp Almond Flour
- 1 tbsp Lakanto Golden Sweetener, or decision of sugar
- 2 tsp Heavy Cream
- 1 tsp Cream Cheese, relaxed
- 1/2 tsp Pumpkin Spice
- 1/2 tsp Baking Powder
- 1/2 tsp Vanilla
- 1 tsp Choczero Maple Syrup or 1/8 tsp Maple Extract

Tasty Keto Pizza Chaffle Recipe

INGREDIENTS

CHAFFLE CRUST

- 1 Egg

- 1/2 cup Mozzarella Cheese
- 1 tsp Coconut Flour
- 1/4 tsp Baking Powder
- 1/8 tsp Garlic Powder
- 1/8 tsp Italian Seasoning
- Pinch of Salt

Pizza Topping

- 1 tbsp Rao's Marinara Sauce
- 1/2 cup Mozzarella Cheese
- 3 Pepperoni's, cut into four
- Shredded Parmesan Cheese, discretionary
- Parsley, discretionary

Best Oreo Keto Chaffles

INGREDIENTS

CHOCOLATE CHAFFLE

- 1 Egg
- 1 1/2 tbsp Unsweetened Cocoa
- 2 tbsp Lakanto Monkfruit, or decision of sugar
- 1 tbsp Heavy Cream
- 1 tsp Coconut Flour
- 1/2 tsp Baking Powder
- 1/2 tsp Vanilla

FILLING

- Whipped Cream (interchange icing formula in notes beneath)

Guidelines

- Preheat mini waffle producer.
- In a small bowl, join all chaffle ingredients.
- Pour a portion of the chaffle blend into the focal point of the waffle iron. Permit to cook for 3-5 minutes.

Keto Peanut Butter Cup Chaffle

INGREDIENTS

CHAFFLE

- 1 Egg
- 1 tbsp Heavy Cream
- 1 tbsp Unsweetened Cocoa
- 1 tbsp Lakanto Powdered Sweetener
- 1 tsp Coconut Flour
- 1/2 tsp Vanilla Extract
- 1/2 Cake Batter Flavor (we utilize this)
- 1/4 tsp Baking Powder

Nutty spread FILLING

- 3 tbsp All regular Peanut Butter
- 2 tsp Lakanto Powdered Sweetener
- 2 tbsp Heavy Cream

Keto Snickerdoodle Chaffle

INGREDIENTS

- 1 Egg
- 1/2 cup Mozzarella Cheese
- 2 tbsp Almond Flour
- 1 tbsp Lakanto Golden Sweetener
- 1/2 tsp Vanilla Extract
- 1/4 tsp Cinnamon
- 1/2 tsp Baking Powder
- 1/4 tsp Cream of tartar, discretionary

Covering

- 1 tbsp Butter
- 2 tbsp Lakanto Classic Sweetener
- 1/2 tsp Cinnamon

Guidelines

- Preheat your mini waffle producer.
- In a little bowl, join all chaffle ingredients.
- Pour a portion of the chaffle blend on to the focal point of the waffle iron. Permit to cook for 3-5 minutes.
- Carefully expel and rehash for the second chaffle. Permit chaffles to cool so they fresh.
- In a little bowl, consolidate sugar and cinnamon for covering.
- Melt spread in a little microwave-safe bowl and brush the chaffles with the margarine.

- Sprinkle sugar and cinnamon blend on the two sides of the chaffles once they're brushed with margarine.

White Bread Keto Chaffle | Wonder Bread Chaffle

INGREDIENTS

- 1 Egg
- 3 tbsp Almond Flour
- 1 tbsp Mayonnaise
- 1/4 tsp Baking Powder
- 1 tsp Water

Guidelines

- Preheat mini waffle producer.
- In a cup, whisk the egg until beaten.
- Add almond flour, mayonnaise, heating powder, and water.
- When the waffle producer is warmed, cautiously pour 1/2 of the hitter in the waffle creator and close the top. Permit to cook for 3-5 minutes.
- Carefully expel from the waffle creator and put in a safe spot for 2-3 minutes to fresh up.
- Repeat directions again for the second chaffle.

Best Oreo Keto Chaffles

INGREDIENTS

CHOCOLATE CHAFFLE

- 1 Egg
- 1 1/2 tbsp Unsweetened Cocoa
- 2 tbsp Lakanto Monkfruit, or decision of sugar
- 1 tbsp Heavy Cream
- 1 tsp Coconut Flour
- 1/2 tsp Baking Powder
- 1/2 tsp Vanilla

FILLING

- Whipped Cream (exchange icing formula in notes beneath)

Guidelines

- Preheat mini waffle producer.
- In a small bowl, join all chaffle ingredients.
- Pour a portion of the chaffle blend into the focal point of the waffle iron. Permit to cook for 3-5 minutes.

Keto Chocolate Chip Chaffle Keto Recipe

Ingredients

- 1 egg
- 1 tbsp substantial whipping cream
- 1/2 tsp coconut flour
- 1 3/4 tsp Lakanto monk fruit brilliant can utilize pretty much to change the sweetness
- 1/4 tsp preparing powder

- pinch of salt
- 1 tbsp Lily's Chocolate Chips

Directions

1. Turn on the waffle creator with the goal that it warms up.
2. In a little bowl, join all ingredients with the exception of the chocolate chips and mix well until consolidated.
3. Grease waffle producer, at that point, pour half of the hitter onto the base plate of the waffle creator.
4. Cook it for 5 minutes or until the chocolate chip chaffle pastry is brilliant dark colored at that point expel from waffle creator with a fork, being mindful so as not to burn your fingers.

Keto Strawberry Cheesecake Shake

INGREDIENTS

- 1 cup Almond Milk, unsweetened
- 2oz Cream cheddar
- 1/2 cup Strawberries
- 2 tbsp Heavy cream
- 1 tbsp Lakanto monk fruit, or decision of sugar
- 1/2 tsp Vanilla
- 1 tbsp ChocZero Strawberry Syrup, discretionary

Directions

1. Add every one of the ingredients into a blender and mix until smooth. Include ice-blocks varying. Appreciate!

Keto Taco Chaffle Recipe (Crispy Taco Shells)

Ingredients

- 1 egg white
- 1/4 cup Monterey jack cheddar, destroyed (stuffed firmly)
- 1/4 cup sharp cheddar, destroyed (stuffed firmly)
- 3/4 tsp water
- 1 tsp coconut flour
- 1/4 tsp preparing powder
- 1/8 tsp stew powder
- pinch of salt

Directions

1. Plug the Dash Mini Waffle Maker in the divider and oil delicately once it is hot.
2. Combine the entirety of the ingredients in a bowl and mix to consolidate.
3. Spoon out 1/2 of the player on the waffle creator and close top. Set a clock for 4 minutes and don't lift the cover until the cooking time is finished. In the event that you do, it will resemble the taco chaffle shell isn't

set up appropriately. However it will. You need to let it cook the whole 4 minutes before lifting the cover.

Maple Pumpkin Keto Waffle Recipe (Chaffle)

Ingredients

- 2 eggs
- 3/4 tsp heating powder
- 2 tsp pumpkin puree (100% pumpkin)
- 3/4 tsp pumpkin pie zest
- 4 tsp substantial whipping cream
- 2 tsp Lakanto Sugar-Free Maple Syrup
- 1 tsp coconut flour
- 1/2 cup mozzarella cheddar, destroyed
- 1/2 tsp vanilla
- pinch of salt

Guidelines

1. Turn on a waffle or chaffle producer. I utilize the Dash Mini Waffle Maker.
2. In a little bowl, join all ingredients.
3. Cover the scramble mini waffle producer with 1/4 of the player and cook for 3-4 minutes.
4. Repeat 3 additional occasions until you have made 4 Maple Syrup Pumpkin Keto Waffles (Chaffles).
5. Serve with without sugar maple syrup or keto frozen yogurt.

Keto Chaffle Breakfast Sandwich

Ingredients

- 1 egg
- 1/2 cup Monterey Jack Cheese
- 1 tablespoon almond flour
- 2 tablespoons spread

Directions

1. In a little bowl, blend the egg, almond flour, and Monterey Jack Cheese.
2. Pour a portion of the hitter into your mini waffle creator and cook for 3-4 minutes. At that point, cook the remainder of the player to make a second chaffle.
3. In a little container, dissolve 2 tablespoons of spread. Include the chaffles and cook each side for 2 minutes. Pushing down while they are cooking gently on the highest point of them, so they are fresh up better.
4. Remove from the container and let sit for 2 minutes.

Mini Keto Pizza Recipe

Ingredients

- 1/2 cup Shredded Mozzarella cheddar
- 1 tablespoon almond flour
- 1/2 tsp heating powder
- 1 egg

- 1/4 tsp garlic powder
- 1/4 tsp basil
- 2 tablespoons low carb pasta sauce
- 2 tablespoons mozzarella cheddar

Guidelines

1. While the waffle producer is warming up, in a bowl blend mozzarella cheddar, preparing powder, garlic, premise, egg, and almond flour.
2. Pour 1/2 the blend into your mini waffle producer.
3. Cook it for 3-5 min. until your pizza waffle is totally cooked. On the off chance that you check it and the waffle adheres to the waffle creator, let it cook for one more moment or two.

Sugar-Free Vanilla Buttercream Frosting

Ingredients

- 1 cup margarine room temperature
- 1.5 cups swerve confectioner
- 2 tbsp Heavy Whipping Cream
- 1 tsp vanilla concentrate

Guidelines

1. Place your margarine and swerve in the bowl of your blender. Combine them on low speed until the sugar is joined.

2. Mix in the substantial cream and the vanilla concentrate.
3. Turn the blender up to medium-fast and keep blending for 6-8 minutes until light and feathery.

Keto Blueberry Chaffle

This scrumptious keto blueberry waffles are, in fact, called a Keto Chaffle! What's more, a kid is it delish! Consummately sweet, with succulent blueberries, these blueberry keto chaffles taste extraordinary and are low carb and keto well disposed.

Ingredients

- 1 cup of mozzarella cheddar
- 2 tablespoons almond flour
- 1 tsp preparing powder
- 2 eggs
- 1 tsp cinnamon
- 2 tsp of Swerve
- 3 tablespoon blueberries

Directions

1. Heat up your Dash mini waffle creator.
2. In a blending bowl include the mozzarella cheddar, almond flour, preparing powder, eggs, cinnamon,

swerve, and blueberries. Blend well, so every one of the ingredients is combined.
3. Spray your mini waffle creator with non-stick cooking splash.
4. Add shortly less than 1/4 a cup of blueberry keto waffle hitter.

Bacon Cheddar Chaffles Recipe

- 1 egg
- 1.2 cup cheddar
- Bacon bits to taste
- Mix and cook until fresh.

Bacon Jalapeno Chaffles Recipe

1. 1/2 cup destroyed swiss/gruyere mix
2. 1 egg
3. 2 tablespoons cooked bacon pieces
4. 1 tablespoon diced crisp jalapenos
5. Cook until fresh. Works incredibly as a bun to a cheeseburger.

Keto Cauliflower Chaffles Recipe

You can make the most delightful keto cauliflower chaffle formula with only a bunch of ingredients and a couple of moments! This formula will be your new top choice!

Ingredients

- 1 cup riced cauliflower
- 1/4 Tbsp. Garlic Powder
- 1/4 Tbsp. Ground Black Pepper
- 1/2 Tbsp. Italian Seasoning
- 1/4 Tbsp. salt
- 1/2 cup destroyed mozzarella cheddar or destroyed Mexican mix cheddar
- 1 Egg
- 1/2 cup destroyed parmesan cheddar

Sandwich Bread Chaffles Recipe

- 1 egg
- 2 tablespoon almond flour
- 1 tablespoon mayo
- 1/8 Tbsp. heating powder
- 1 Tbsp. water
- Sweetener and garlic powder (discretionary)
- Makes 2 chaffles, and you can undoubtedly slice them down the middle for a bun.

Sweet Chaffles Recipes

To make chaffles sweet, the conceivable outcomes are inestimable! You can just utilize the base formula and include some Keto-accommodating sugars.

In the event that you need to include some sweet seasoning after, you can sprinkle a wide range of Keto-accommodating magnificence on top. I like to utilize this Lakanto Maple Syrup. Something else, on the off chance that you need more than that, you can use the recipes beneath!

Chocolate Brownie Chaffles

- Making the Keto Chocolate Brownies Batter.
- Stir and pour in the mini waffle producer.
- You can see the entire formula and a video here for how to make chocolate chaffles
- Cook 5-7 minutes until firm. – TwoSleevers

Mint Chocolate Broffle (Brownie Waffle)

- Use this keto brownie formula.
- Add hacked walnuts, and each broffle (brownie waffle) utilized 3 tablespoons of player for 7 min.
- The formula for the buttercream depends on Urvashi's maple walnut buttercream formula, just with mint rather than maple separate.

Lemon Pound Cake Chaffles

Numerous individuals are cutting my lemon pound cake formula by 1/4 and making Cake Chaffles out of them.

Crusty fruit-filled treat CHAFFLES

- 1.2 cup mozzarella cheddar
- 1 egg

- Add the mozzarella to the waffle producer.
- Put the egg on top.
- Sprinkle on crusty fruit-filled treat zest and 5 sugar-free chocolate chips.
- Serve with margarine on top.

Cream Cheese Carrot Cake Chaffles

- 2 tablespoons cream cheddar or a blend of 1 tablespoon cream cheddar and 2 tablespoons destroyed mozzarella cheddar
- 1/2 pat of margarine
- 1 tablespoon finely destroyed carrot
- 1 tablespoon of sugar of your decision. I utilized Splenda.
- 1 tablespoon almond flour
- 1 Tbsp. pumpkin pie zest
- 1/2 Tbsp. vanilla
- 1/2 Tbsp. heating powder
- 1 egg
- OPTIONAL

I included 6 raisins, 1 tablespoon of destroyed coconut, and 1/2 tablespoon of pecans to the blender ingredients.

Cream Cheese Frosting

- 1 tablespoon cream cheddar
- 1 pat spread

- 1 Tbsp. sugar of decision. I utilized Cinnamon Brown Sugar without sugar syrup.
- Heat up, waffle creator. I utilized a mini Dash. I oiled with a silicon brush dunked in coconut oil.
- Microwave cream cheddar, mozzarella, and spread for 15 seconds to liquefy the cheeses to make consolidating simpler. I did this in an enchantment slug cup to mix.
- Add the remainder of the chaffle ingredients to the blender cup and mix until smooth and consolidated.
- Add a player to a waffle creator. For the Dash, I included 2 stacking tablespoons, and it made 3 chaffles.
- While making the chaffle, heat up the spread and cream cheddar for the icing. Blend until smooth, and consolidate your sugar. Sprinkle over chaffles as wanted.

Cinnamon Chaffles

- 1/2 cup mozzarella
- 1 egg
- 1 tbsp vanilla concentrate
- 1/2 tsp preparing powder
- 1 tbsp almond flour
- Sprinkle of cinnamon
- Mix together and cook until chaffles are firm.

Cinnamon Swirl Chaffles

- CHAFFLE:
- 1 oz cream cheddar, mollified
- 1 huge egg, beaten
- 1 tsp vanilla concentrate
- 1 tbsp almond flour, superfine
- 1 tbsp Splenda
- 1 tsp cinnamon
- ICING:
- 1 oz cream cheddar, mollified
- 1 tbsp. spread, unsalted
- 1 tbsp Splenda
- 1/2 tsp vanilla

Cinnamon Drizzle:

- 1/2 tbsp spread
- 1 tbsp Splenda
- 1 tsp cinnamon
- Heat up waffle creator, and I brushed on coconut oil on my DASH.
- Stir up the chaffle ingredients until smooth.
- Utilize a spoon to include 2 piling tbsp of the player to the waffle iron. It will make 3 little waffles.
- Cook to your ideal waffle freshness. I did 4 min. They resembled a delicate waffle.

- Cool on a rack.
- Mix the icing and cinnamon shower in little dishes. Warmth in the microwave for 10 secs to find a workable pace consistency. Whirl on cooled waffles.

Greek Marinated Feta And Olives

Ingredients

- 1 cup olive oil
- 1/4 Tbsp. oregano
- 1/4 Tbsp. thyme
- 1/2 Tbsp. dried rosemary
- 1 cup kalamata olives
- 1 cup of green olives
- 1/2 pound feta

Directions

- In a little pot heat, the oil, oregano, thyme, rosemary together over medium warmth for 5 minutes to imbue the oil with the herbs.
- Set the oil to the side and enable it to cool for 15 minutes.
- Cut the feta into 1/2 inch 3D shapes.

Air Fryer Peanut Chicken

Not many things state "Thai food" like Peanut Chicken. This Peanut Chicken formula takes the dish to an unheard-of level and is effectively made in your air fryer!

Ingredients

- 1 pound Bone-in Skin-on Chicken Thighs
- For the Sauce
- 1/4 cup Creamy Peanut Butter
- 1 tablespoon Sriracha Sauce, (modify for your zest needs)
- 1 tablespoon Soy Sauce
- 2 tablespoons sweet chili sauce
- 2 tablespoons lime juice
- 1 Tbsp. Minced Garlic
- 1 Tbsp. minced ginger
- 1/2 Tbsp. salt, to taste
- 1/2 cup high temp water

Green Beans With Bacon

Right now, Pot Green Beans with Bacon formula is a fast, low carb, and nutritious dish that can be eaten either as a side dish or as a low carb dinner. Just beans, bacon, and a couple of seasonings make this a quick and simple dish.

Ingredients

- 1 cup (160 g) onion, diced

- 5 cuts (5 cuts) Bacon, diced
- 6 cups (660 g) green beans, cut in

Keto Buffalo Chicken Casserole

This Buffalo Chicken Casserole is as flavorful filling dish with the perfect measure of kick! It's the ideal weeknight supper that requires little exertion to make.

Ingredients

- 4 cups rotisserie chicken, destroyed
- 1/2 cup Onion, slashed
- 1/4 cup Cream
- 1/4 cup hot wing sauce
- 1/4 cup blue cheddar, disintegrated
- 2 ounces Cream Cheese, diced
- pepper
- 1/4 cup Green Onions, slashed

German Red Cabbage

Appreciate this customary German Red Cabbage formula made in a non-conventional way! Make this wonderfully prepared side dish directly in your Instant Pot!

Ingredients

- 6 cups red cabbage, cleaved
- 3 Granny Smith Apples, little, cut 1 inch thick
- 2 tablespoons liquefied margarine, or oil

- 1/3 cup Apple Cider Vinegar
- 2-3 tablespoons Sugar
- 1 Tbsp. salt
- 1/2 Tbsp. Ground Black Pepper
- 1/4 Tbsp. Ground Cloves
- 2 sound leaves

Maple Pecan Bars With Sea Salt

Ingredients

For the Crust

- Non-Stick Spray
- 1/3 cup Butter, mellowed
- 1/4 cup Brown Sugar, immovably stuffed
- 1 cup All-Purpose Flour
- 1/4 Kosher tea Salt

For the Filling

- 4 TBS Butter (1/2 stick), diced
- 1/2 cup Brown Sugar
- 1/4 cup Pure Maple Syrup
- 1/4 cup Whole Milk
- 1/4 tea Vanilla concentrate

Moment POT VEGETARIAN CHILI

Ingredients

- 1 cup Onion, cleaved

- 1 cup Canned Fire Roasted Tomatoes
- 1.5 tablespoons Minced Garlic
- 3 corn tortillas
- 1 tablespoon Chipotle Chile in Adobo Sauce, cleaved
- 1 tablespoon Mexican Red Chili Powder, (not cayenne)
- 2 Tbsp.s Ground Cumin
- 2 Tbsp.s salt
- 1 Tbsp. Dried Oregano
- 1 cup Water
- 1/2 cup dried pinto beans, doused medium-term or for 1 hour in heated water
- 1/2 cup dried dark beans, splashed medium-term or for 1 hour in high temp water
- 2 cups corn, new or defrosted solidified corn
- 2 cups zucchini, hacked

Keto Almendrados Cookies | Spanish Almond Keto Cookies

Ingredients

- 1.5 cups Superfine Almond Flour
- 1/2 cup Swerve
- 1 huge Egg
- 1 Tbsp. Lemon Extract
- 1 tablespoon lemon get-up-and-go
- 24 whitened almonds

Directions

1. In a medium bowl, beat egg. Include almond flour, swerve and lemon and combine to make a strong mixture. Cover and refrigerate for 1-2 hours.
2. Preheat stove to 350 degrees. Line a heating sheet with material paper.
3. Pinching off bits of batter about the size of a pecan, fold them into balls.

Keto Taco

Prep. time: 11 minutes/Cook time: 20 minutes/Serves 3

Need to begin the day surprising? Morning keto is such an astounding beginning to a delightful day. Light and superb with a lot of splendid hues and feelings.

8 oz. Mozzarella cheddar, destroyed; 6 Eggs, enormous 2 tbsp. Margarine

3 Bacon stripes ½ Avocado 1 oz. Cheddar, destroyed Pepper and salt to taste

Keto Omelet With Goat Cheese And Spinach

Prep. time: 5 minutes

3 Large eggs 1 Medium green onion 1 oz. Goat cheddar ¼ Onion

2 tbsp. Margarine 2 cups Spinach 2 tbsp. Substantial cream Salt and pepper to taste

Chicken And Cheese Quesadilla

Prep. time: 10 minutes/Serves 4

For capsules: 6 Eggs 4 oz. Coconut flour 6 oz. Substantial cream ½ tsp. Thickener Pink salt and pepper 1 tbsp. Olive oil for fricasseeing

For the quesadilla: 4 oz. Cheddar destroyed 8 oz. Chicken bosom cooked and destroyed 1 tbsp. Parsley, cleaved (discretionary)

Gluten Free Sports Nutrition Basics

At the point when you're a competitor, it's imperative to get a decent assortment of protein, sugars, and sound fats for the duration of the day. Evading gluten implies picking gluten-free nourishments and wiping out wheat, grain, and rye items from your eating routine to keep away from aggravation, swelling, stomach torment, cramps, looseness of the bowels, exhaustion, lack of healthy sustenance, iron deficiency, and blockage.

Protein Needs

The American College of Sports Medicine and the Academy of Nutrition and Dietetics prescribe athletes eat 0.5 to 0.8 grams of protein per pound of their body weight day by day, and 15 to 20 percent of their complete calories from protein.

Pick a lot of protein-rich nourishments, for example,

- Lean meats, poultry, fish, and fish
- Eggs
- Low-fat dairy nourishments or dairy substitutes
- Tofu or other soy items
- Legumes
- Nuts, seeds, and nut margarines

Carb Requirements

Carbs are essential for athletes since this macronutrient is a competitor's primary vitality source. Athletes get 50 to 60 percent of their calories from carbs, or 2.7 to 4.6 grams of carbs per pound of body weight day by day. Pick sound, gluten-free carbs, for example,

- Gluten-free oats, oats, and oats (must indicate gluten-free)
- Rice
- Quinoa
- Fruits
- Starchy vegetables like potatoes, yams, peas, corn, and vegetables

Fat Recommendations

Dietary fat should make up around 20 to 30 percent of a competitor's calorie consumption. Pick sound fats, for example,

- Nuts and seeds
- Nut margarines
- Plant-based oils
- Avocadoes
- Olives

Gluten Free Recipes for Athletes

Gluten Free Recipes For Athletes

The accompanying gluten-free recipes make certain to be a hit with athletes, regardless of whether utilized before working out for a snappy increase in vitality or as a post-practice recuperation feast or bite.

Almond Blast Protein Shake

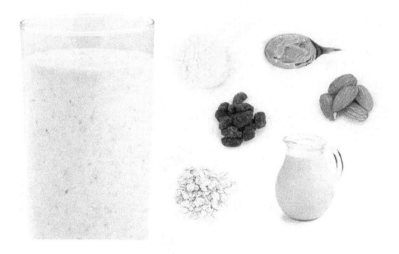

This shake assists athletes with devouring protein, which is basic for muscle improvement.

Fixings

- 2 scoops of gluten-free vanilla-seasoned protein powder
- 1.5 cups of low-fat milk, soy milk, or almond milk
- ½ cup of gluten-free oats

- ½ cup of raisins
- 12 fragmented almonds
- 1 tablespoon of nutty spread

Bearings

Mix all fixings together in blender and serve chilled.

Chocolate Peanut Butter Protein Balls

Anoth er protein-rich formula, these protein balls make an incredible pre-or post-exercise nibble.

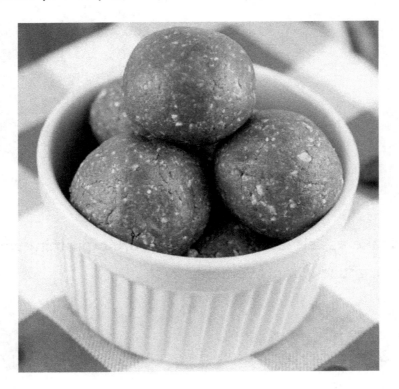

Fixings

- 1 cup of gluten-free moved oats

- 1/2 cup of characteristic nutty spread
- 1/3 cup of nectar
- 2 tablespoons of flax seeds
- 2 tablespoons of chia seeds
- 1 tablespoon of gluten-free chocolate protein powder

Bearings

1. Stir all fixings together in a bowl.
2. Cover the bowl with cling wrap.
3. Refrigerate blend for 30 minutes.
4. Scoop chilled blend into balls and serve.

Tomato Spinach Omelet

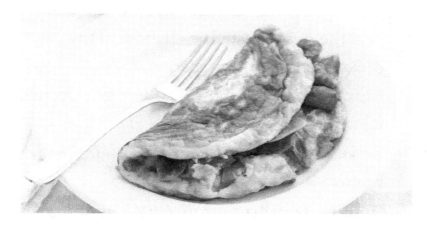

With sound protein and nutrient-thick veggies, this formula is an extraordinary method to begin the day.

Fixings

- 4 enormous eggs
- 1/2 cup broiler cooked tomatoes

- 1 cup infant spinach leaves
- 1/2 cup feta cheddar
- 1 tablespoon olive oil

Headings

1. Saute the spinach and tomatoes in the olive oil over medium-low warmth for a few minutes.
2. Pour the beaten eggs into the skillet and gradually shake to circulate equitably all through.
3. After around two minutes, slacken the omelet blend from the base of the container to forestall staying.
4. Sprinkle the feta cheddar over the omelet.
5. Fold the omelet with the cheddar in the center and cook until it is brilliant darker.
6. Flip the omelet and cook for one increasingly minute.
7. Serve with gluten-free toast and orange cuts, whenever wanted.

Quinoa And Asparagus Chicken Salad

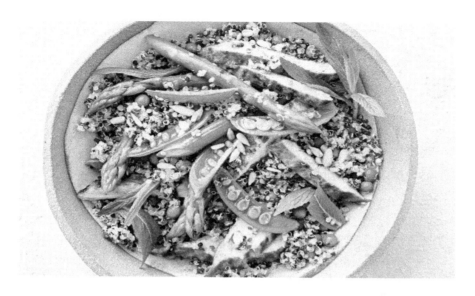

This formula is an extraordinary wellspring of gluten-free complex carbs and protein.

Fixings

- 1/2 cup uncooked quinoa
- 2 ounces chicken bosom
- 1/2 cup sun-dried tomatoes
- 10-ounces asparagus
- 1/2 cup feta cheddar
- 1 tablespoon olive oil
- Salt and pepper

Headings

1. Cook the quinoa as guided and add it to an enormous bowl.

2. Steam the asparagus for around 5 minutes and cut it into little pieces.
3. Add the asparagus, tomatoes, feta cheddar, and chicken bosom to bowl with the quinoa.
4. Add the olive oil, salt, and pepper.
5. Mix all fixings and appreciate!

Turkey Chili

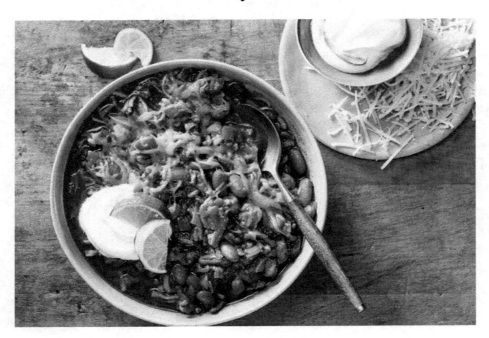

Lean protein, complex carbs, and bunches of flavor makes this a thought formula for athletes.

Fixings

- 2 cups water
- 1 pound ground turkey

- 1 jar of diced tomatoes
- 1 jar of kidney beans
- 1 slashed onion
- 1 1/2 Tbsp.s olive oil
- 1 tablespoon minced garlic
- 2 tablespoons bean stew powder
- 1/2 Tbsp. oregano
- 1/2 Tbsp. ground cumin
- 1/2 Tbsp. paprika
- Salt and pepper to taste

Headings

1. Cook the turkey and olive oil in a pot over medium warmth until darker.
2. Add the onions and cook until delicate.
3. Add the rest of the fixings and heat the blend to the point of boiling.
4. Reduce the warmth to low and stew for about 30 minutes.

Anti-Aging Recipes

Edamame With Ground Bonito And Seaweed

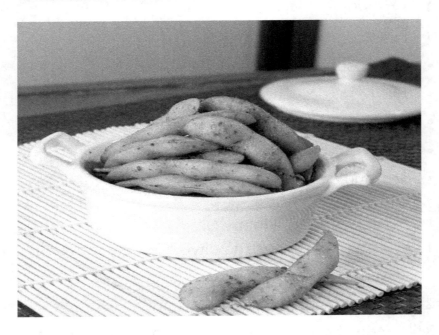

- PREP TIME: 5 MINUTES
- COOK TIME: 6 MINUTES
- TOTAL TIME: 11 MINUTES
- CATEGORY: SNACK
- CUISINE: VEGETARIAN

Fixings

- 1 pound edamame (new or solidified)
- 1/4 nori sheet
- 2 tablespoons bonito chips
- 1/2 Tbsp. salt

Directions

1. Follow bearings on edamame bundle on how to cook them (I lean toward bubbling them two or three minutes not as much as what the headings state, as it makes them less soft). Channel them and let them dry for 2-3 minutes.
2. Break the nori and add it to an espresso/flavor processor alongside the bonito pieces and the salt. Granulate the blend until it nearly transforms into a powder.
3. Put the edamame in a blending bowl and sprinkle the powdered blend over them. Hurl a couple of times and serve.

Korean Pickles

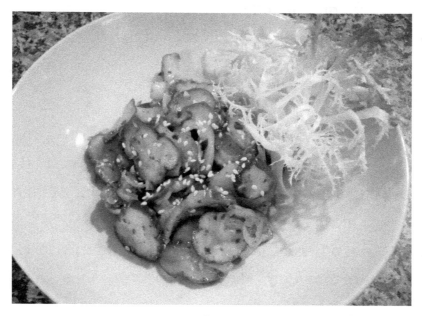

- PREP TIME: 10 MINUTES
- COOK TIME: 15 MINUTES
- TOTAL TIME: 25 MINUTES
- CATEGORY: CONDIMENT
- CUISINE: KOREAN

Fixings

- 2 cups daikon (stripped and julienned (cut into little strips))
- 1 medium carrot (stripped and julienned)
- 1 shallot (finely hacked)
- 2 tablespoons water
- 3 tablespoons rice vinegar
- 2 Tbsp.s tobanjan (Korean stew glue)
- 2 Tbsp.s sesame oil
- 1 Tbsp. granulated sugar
- 2 Tbsp.s salt (in addition to included 1/2 Tbsp.)
- 1 tablespoon sesame seeds

Directions

1. Put the daikon, carrots and shallot in a medium size blending bowl and include 2 tsp salt. Rapidly blend in with your hands and leave for 10 minutes, to mollify the veggies.
2. In a different little bowl, blend water, rice vinegar and tobanjan. Mix until tobanjan has weakened

and include sugar, 1/2 tsp salt, and sesame oil. Mix well until sugar and salt have dissolved.
3. Rinse the vegetable, channel and press out overabundance water. Return the vegetable in the blending bowl and pour the tobanjan blend over.
4. Add sesame seeds and utilizing chopsticks or a spoon, blend until veggies are all around covered. Serve or let pickle for as long as 3 days.

Nourishment

- Calories: 233
- Saturated Fat: 2

Pan Fried Food Beef With Spicy Hoisin Sauce

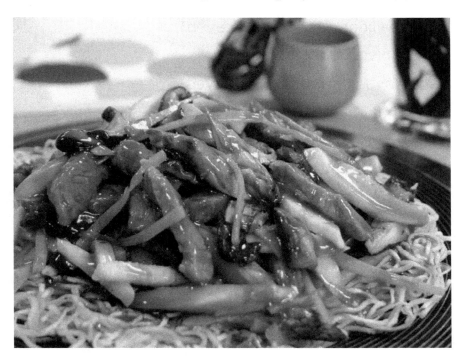

Make this hot, valid Szechuan hoisin pan sear hamburger formula in under 20 minutes!

- PREP TIME: 10 MINUTES
- COOK TIME: 6 MINUTES
- TOTAL TIME: 16 MINUTES
- YIELD: 2 PEOPLE 1X
- CATEGORY: MAIN
- CUISINE: CHINESE

Fixings

- 1/2 pound lean meat (meagerly cut scaled down)
- 1 red chime pepper (center and seeded, cut into meager strips (julienne))
- 4 scallions (generally cleaved)
- 1 tablespoon vegetable oil
- 2 cloves garlic (finely cleaved)
- 2 Thai bean stews (finely slashed)
- 2 tablespoons hoisin sauce
- 1 Tbsp. white miso glue
- For the marinade:
- 1 tablespoon dull soy
- 1 tablespoon soy sauce
- 1 tablespoon shaoxing wine or dry sherry
- 1 tablespoon corn starch

Directions

1. Put all the element for the marinade in a bowl with the meat. Blend well and put in a safe spot for 30 minutes.
2. In a medium size container over high warmth, include oil, garlic and chiles and cook for 1 moment.
3. Add meat and cook for 3 minutes.
4. Add pepper and scallions and cook for 2 minutes, mixing regularly.
5. Turn the warmth off, include hoisin sauce and miso glue, mix well until glue has broken up. Serve pan sear with white rice.

NOTES

This Stir Fry Beef With Hoisin Sauce:

Exceptionally high in iron

High in selenium

Extremely high in nutrient B6

Extremely high in nutrient B12

Extremely high in nutrient C

High in zinc

Sauteed Kale With Mustard Sauce

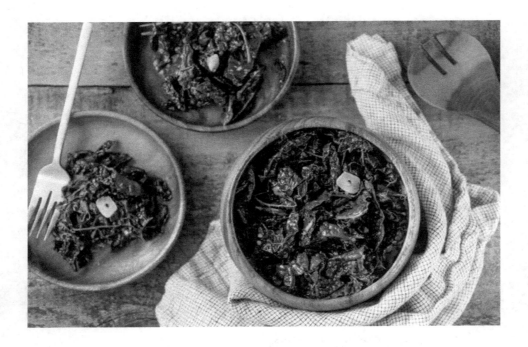

- PREP TIME: 5 MINUTES
- COOK TIME: 7 MINUTES
- TOTAL TIME: 12 MINUTES
- YIELD: 2 1X
- CATEGORY: SIDE

Fixings

- 2 tablespoons additional virgin olive oil
- 1 clove garlic (minced)
- 1/4 cup white wine
- 1 pack kale (ribs expelled and finely hacked)
- 1/2 Tbsp. genuine salt
- 1/4 Tbsp. ground dark pepper
- 1 Tbsp. dijon mustard

- 1/4 cup milk

Directions

1. In a container over medium/high warmth, include olive oil and garlic. Cook for 1 moment.
2. Add white wine, mix well and cook for 1 moment.
3. Add kale, mix well and cook for 4 minutes, mixing continually.
4. Add salt and pepper, mix and cook for 1 moment.
5. Turn off the warmth, include milk and dijon mustard and rapidly mix until fluid is no more. Serve.

Sauteed Green Beans With Chilies

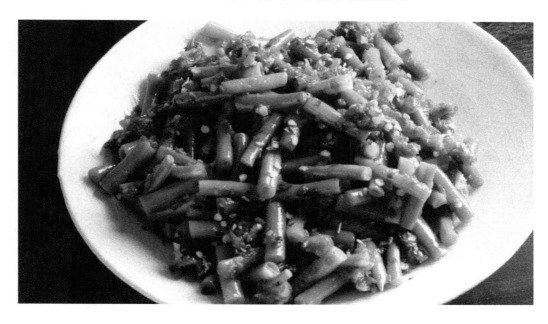

- PREP TIME: 10 MINUTES
- COOK TIME: 5 MINUTES
- TOTAL TIME: 15 MINUTES
- YIELD: 4 1X
- CATEGORY: SIDE
- CUISINE: CHINESE

Fixings

- 2 cloves garlic (finely hacked)
- 1 Tbsp. ginger (stripped and finely hacked)
- 1 pound green beans (washed)
- 2 tablespoons vegetable oil
- 1 Tbsp. dried red chilies (hacked)
- 1 tablespoon shellfish sauce
- 1 tablespoon soy sauce
- 1 Tbsp. sesame oil

Directions

1. Bring a pot of salted water to bubble (not as salty as the ocean, yet enough that you can taste it).
2. Meanwhile, flush and cut the parts of the bargains bean.
3. When water is bubbling, whiten the green beans for 3 minutes. Channel.

4. In a medium size container, include the vegetable oil, garlic, ginger and dried chilies. Cook for a moment and include green beans.
5. Toss and cook for one more moment, at that point include soy sauce and clam sauce.
6. Toss well, include sesame oil and turn the warmth off. Serve.

Nourishment

- Calories: 109
- Saturated Fat: 1

Shrimp And Celery Salad With Wasabi Mayo

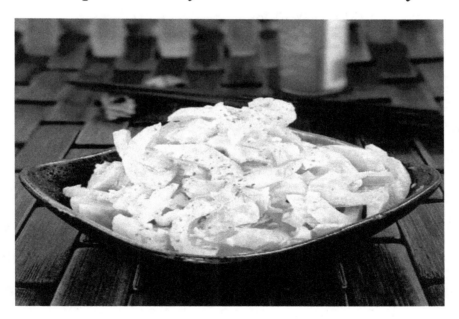

Rich, crunchy and

- PREP TIME: 10 MINUTES

- COOK TIME: 5 MINUTES
- TOTAL TIME: 15 MINUTES
- YIELD: 4 SIDES 1X
- CATEGORY: SALADS
- METHOD: CHOPPING
- CUISINE: JAPANESE

Fixings

- 16–20 huge crude shrimps, deveined and stripped
- 3 celery stalks, cleaved reduced down
- 2 tablespoon orange, red or green chime peppers, diced
- 1/4 cup mayonnaise
- 1/2 tablespoon rice vinegar
- 1/2 Tbsp. wasabi glue
- Salt and ichimi togarashi to taste

Directions

1. Bring a little pot of water with 1 tablespoon salt to bubble.
2. Add celery and heat up (this procedure is called whitening) for 2 minutes. Channel and wash celery in cool water. Put in a safe spot.
3. Bring another little pot of water to bubble, include shrimps and bubble for 3 minutes. Channel, wash in chilly water and put in a safe spot.

4. In a medium size blending bowl, mix mayonnaise, rice vinegar and wasabi glue together until smooth.
5. Dry the shrimps with a paper towel or hand towel, and slash them into reduced down. Add to the blending bowl.
6. Add celery and ringer peppers to the blending bowl, and mix the entirety of the fixings well. Season with salt and pepper. Serve cold.

NOTES

This shrimp and celery serving of mixed greens will keep refrigerated in a hermetically sealed compartment for as long as 2 days.

Fish Steak With Tomato Relish

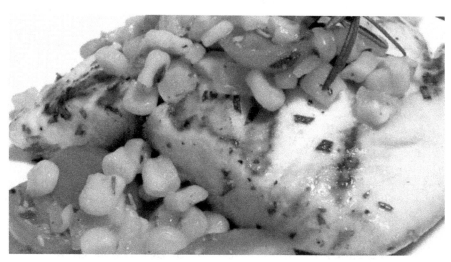

- PREP TIME: 5 MINUTES
- COOK TIME: 17 MINUTES

- TOTAL TIME: 22 MINUTES
- YIELD: 2 1X
- CATEGORY: MAIN
- CUISINE: FISH, SEAFOOD

Fixings

- 2 pounds fish steak
- 3 tablespoons additional virgin olive oil
- 1 clove garlic (finely hacked)
- 1 half quart treasure or cherry tomatoes (finely hacked)
- 1/2 medium onion (finely hacked)
- 8 leaves new basil (generally hacked)
- 1 Tbsp. sugar
- salt and pepper to taste
- lemon wedges (to serve)

Directions

1. In a dish over high warmth, include 2 tbsp olive oil, garlic and onions, and cook for 3-4 minutes, until onions are translucent. Include tomatoes and sugar, and cook for 5 minutes, or until the blend is practically similar to a sauce. Mood killer the warmth, include basil and season with salt, and pepper.

2. Use a different dish to cook the fish. Season the fish with salt and pepper on the two sides. Hold up until the dish is hot and include the staying 1 tbsp olive oil. Include fish steaks and lower the warmth to medium/high. Spread and cook until all around done (around 7 minutes). Covering the dish keeps the fish clammy, I utilize this stunt for fish, chicken and even meat; it has exactly the intended effect.

Nourishment

- Calories: 655
- Saturated Fat: 4

Stout Vegetable Soup

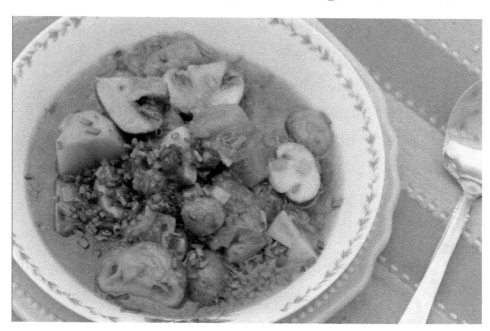

- PREP TIME: 15 MINUTES

- COOK TIME: an hour
- TOTAL TIME: 75 MINUTES
- YIELD: 4 PEOPLE 1X
- CATEGORY: SOUP
- CUISINE: VEGETARIAN

SCALE 1x2x3x

Fixings

- 3 cloves garlic (finely hacked)
- 1 onion (finely hacked)
- 3 tablespoons additional virgin olive oil
- 3 medium carrots (generally cleaved)
- 2 stalks celery (generally cleaved)
- 2 turnips (generally cleaved)
- 1/4 head cabbage (generally cleaved)
- 28 oz can squashed tomatoes
- 7 cups vegetable stock
- 1/2 Tbsp. dried thyme
- dried herbs like basil oregano as well as parsley
- salt and pepper (to taste)

Directions

1. In a huge pot over high warmth, include oil, garlic, dried thyme and onions. Cook for 4-6 minutes until onions relax and turn out to be clear. Include the squashed tomatoes and mix. Include everything

else; carrots, celery, turnips, cabbage, vegetable juices and dried herbs. Season with somewhat salt and bring to bubble.
2. Bring to bubble, spread and lower warmth to a stew. Cook for 25 minutes or until vegetables are cooked through. Keep an eye on your soup on occasion and mix to ensure veggies aren't consuming at the base of the pot.
3. Season with salt and pepper and serve.

NOTES

This stout vegetable soup can likewise be presented with new cleaved parsley and wafers.

CPSIA information can be obtained
at www.ICGtesting.com
Printed in the USA
LVHW101146191120
672145LV00012B/489